GERD DIET COOKBOOK

Delicious Low-Acidity Recipes For Acid Reflux Relief, Heartburn Management, And Digestive Health

DR ELIAN GRIFFIN

Copyright © [Elian Griffin] [2024]. All rights reserved.

Without the publisher's prior written consent, no portion of this publication may be copied, distributed, or transmitted in any way, including by photocopying, recording, or other mechanical or electronic means, with the exception of brief quotations used in all critical reviews.

DISCLAIMER

The nutritional recommendations and recipes in this book are meant solely for informative reasons. They are not meant to replace the counsel, diagnosis, or care of a qualified medical expert. If you have any doubts about a medical condition or dietary requirements, you should always see your physician or another trained healthcare expert.

All reasonable efforts have been taken by the author and publisher to ensure that the information contained in this book is correct as of the date of publication. Recommendations may alter, though, as medical knowledge is always changing. When using any of the recipes or instructions found here, the user assumes all liability and assumes no risk, whether personal or otherwise. People who have certain dietary requirements or medical issues should speak with a healthcare provider for personalized guidance. The given recipes are only ideas; you may need to adjust them to suit your own nutritional needs, tastes, and tolerances.

When you use this book, you agree to release the publisher, the author, and their representatives from any liability for any claims, damages, liabilities, costs, or expenditures resulting from your use of the book.

TABLE OF CONTENTS

CHAPTER ONE 11
GERD DIET INTRODUCTION 11
GERD OVERVIEW 11
IMPORTANCE FOR GERD DIET MANAGEMENT 12
ESSENTIAL GUIDELINES FOR THE GERD DIET 14

CHAPTER TWO 17
FOUNDATIONS OF DIET AND GERD 17
AN OVERVIEW OF SYMPTOMS OF GERD 17
DIETARY INTERVENTIONS FOR GERD 18
FOODS NOT TO EAT TO TREAT GERD 19
FOODS THAT REDUCE THE SYMPTOMS OF GERD 20
OVERVIEW OF GERD-FRIENDLY COOKING METHODS 21

CHAPTER THREE 23
MEAL PLANNING FOR GERD Diet 23
EVALUATING YOUR EXISTING DIET 23
DEVELOPING OBJECTIVES FOR YOUR GERD DIET 24
STRATEGIES FOR MEAL PLANNING 25
PLANNING BALANCED MEALS THAT ARE GERD-FRIENDLY: 26
TIPS FOR GROCERY BUYING WITH GERD-FRIENDLY 26

RECIPES FOR BREAKFAST 28
IDEAS FOR GERD-FRIENDLY BREAKFASTS 28
EASY BREAKFAST RECIPES TO FOLLOW 29
SIMPLE AND QUICK MORNING MEALS 29
HEALTHY SMOOTHIE RECIPE IDEAS 30

- BREAKFAST'S CRITICAL ROLE IN GERD MANAGEMENT 31
- RECIPES FOR LUNCH AND DINNER 33
  - GERD-SAFE SNACKS FOR LUNCH AND DINNER 33
  - APPETIZING AND FILLING MAIN COURSES 33
  - VEGETABLE-BASED RECIPES TO ALLEVIATE GERD 34
  - COOKING TECHNIQUES TO LESSEN GERD SYMPTOMS 35
  - GERD-FRIENDLY SEASONINGS AND FLAVORFUL SAUCES 36
- DESSERTS & SNACKS 37
  - SNACK OPTIONS THAT ARE GOOD FOR GERD PATIENTS 37
  - SWEETS THAT WON'T MAKE YOUR GERD SYMPTOMS 38
  - ENERGIZING SNACK IDEAS 39
  - DESSERTS THAT DON'T AGGRAVATE GERD 39
  - TIPS FOR PORTION CONTROL IN SNACKING 40
- DRINKS AND BEVERAGES 42
  - RECOGNIZING GERD-FRIENDLY DRINKS 42
  - TIPS FOR HYDRATION FOR PEOPLE WITH GERD 43
  - TEAS MADE WITH HERBS TO REDUCE GERD SYMPTOMS 44
  - STEER CLEAR OF TRIGGERING DRINKS 45
  - MAKING COOL DRINKS WITHOUT CAFFEINE OR CITRUS 46
- CHAPTER FOUR 47
  - HANDLING GERD IN PARTICULAR CIRCUMSTANCES 47
    - GERD AND EATING OUT: STRATEGIES AND ADVICE 47
    - TRAVELING WHILE KEEPING YOUR GERD DIET IN CHECK 48
    - GET-TOGETHERS AND GERD-FRIENDLY DECISIONS 49
    - HOW TO CELEBRATE AND HANDLE HOLIDAYS 50

- HANDLING GERD IN HIGH-STRESS SITUATIONS 51
- CHAPTER FIVE 53
  - LIFESTYLE SUGGESTIONS TO REDUCE GERD 53
    - THE VALUE OF EXERCISE IN THE MANAGEMENT OF GERD 53
    - STRATEGIES FOR STRESS REDUCTION IN GERD PATIENTS 54
    - GERD AND SLEEP HYGIENE 55
    - KEEPING A HEALTHY WEIGHT TO MANAGE GERD 56
    - DAILY ROUTINES TO ENCOURAGE GERD-FREE LIVING 58
- CHAPTER SIX 61
  - RECIPES FOR PARTICULAR EVENTS 61
    - RECIPES FOR PARTIES AND GATHERINGS THAT ARE GERD-FRIENDLY 61
    - HOLIDAY MENUS THAT DON'T MAKE YOUR GERD WORSE 62
    - PREPARING FOOD FOR VISITORS WITH GERD CONCERNS 63
    - ENJOYING YOURSELF WITHOUT LOSING YOUR DIET 64
    - DESSERT IDEAS FOR SPECIAL OCCASIONS THAT WON'T SET OFF 64
- CHAPTER SEVEN 67
  - COMMON QUESTIONS AND CONCERNS 67
    - CONTROLLING GERD SYMPTOMS WITHOUT MEDICATIONS 67
    - HANDLING EPISODES OF GERD 68
    - LONG-TERM GERD MANAGEMENT TECHNIQUES 69
    - TIPS FOR PATIENTS WITH RECENTLY DIAGNOSED GERD 70
    - FREQUENTLY ASKED QUESTIONS REGARDING THE DIET FOR 72

ABOUT THE BOOK

The "GERD Diet Cookbook" is a vital resource for anyone attempting to manage their symptoms of gastroesophageal reflux disease (GERD) with food. It provides readers with information on GERD, its symptoms, and how important diet is in controlling symptoms. By emphasizing GERD-friendly dietary principles, the book equips readers with useful methods for reducing symptoms and enhancing their quality of life in general.

Emphasizing foods to avoid that exacerbate symptoms and those that can help mitigate discomfort, the book takes a comprehensive approach to the GERD diet. Its structured chapters teach readers how to effectively plan their GERD diet, from assessing current eating habits to creating balanced meals that support digestive health. This nuanced understanding is complemented by insightful tips on GERD-friendly cooking techniques, ensuring that meals are both nutritious and soothing.

The cookbook is filled with recipes that are specifically crafted to be easy on the stomach while still being delicious and filling. From nutritious smoothies for breakfast to vegetable-based lunch and dinner entrees to inventive snacks and desserts that steer clear of common triggers, the recipes are sure to please a wide range of palates and dietary requirements.

Beyond recipes, the book covers useful lifestyle modifications that support dietary changes, like the value of exercise, stress reduction methods, and improving sleep hygiene—all essential components in effectively managing GERD. Specific scenarios like eating out, traveling, and navigating social gatherings are also covered, giving readers tips on how to stick to a consistent diet in a variety of contexts.

To provide readers with comprehensive support and give them the tools they need to take control of their health, the book includes a section devoted to common concerns and frequently asked questions (FAQs). It covers topics like how to manage symptoms without medication, deal with flare-ups, and provide guidance for those who have just received a diagnosis.

For those seeking to proactively treat GERD through dietary and lifestyle changes, the "GERD Diet Cookbook" proves to be an invaluable resource as it not only focuses on recipes but also offers practical advice for common problems and comprehensive lifestyle improvements.

CHAPTER ONE

GERD DIET INTRODUCTION

GERD OVERVIEW

The chronic digestive disorder known as gastroesophageal reflux disease (GERD) is characterized by the reflux of stomach acid into the esophagus, resulting in symptoms such as heartburn, regurgitation, and discomfort.

The condition is caused by abnormal relaxation or weakening of the lower esophageal sphincter (LES), a muscle that acts as a valve between the esophagus and the stomach, allowing acidic stomach contents to flow backward into the esophagus. If left untreated, this condition can lead to irritation and inflammation of the esophageal lining and may even cause complications.

Comprehending Gastroesophageal reflux disease (GERD) entails identifying its causative agents and manifestations, which can vary from person to person.

Common causative agents include specific foods (such as oily or spicy foods), drinks (such as coffee or alcohol), and lifestyle choices (such as obesity or smoking). Symptoms of GERD include regurgitation of food or sour liquid, difficulty swallowing, persistent coughing, or hoarseness. Diagnosing Gastroenta usually entails a combination of symptom assessment, review of medical history, and diagnostic tests (such as endoscopy or pH monitoring).

Effective management of gastroesophageal reflux disease (GERD) is essential for avoiding complications and enhancing quality of life. Medications, proton pump inhibitors, H2-receptor antagonists, and, in extreme situations, surgery are common treatment approaches. Dietary changes are a major component of symptom management, as they minimize acid reflux and ease symptoms.

IMPORTANCE FOR GERD DIET MANAGEMENT

Dietary management is essential for managing symptoms of gastroreflux disease (GERD) and lowering the frequency of reflux episodes. The main objective of a GERD diet is to minimize acid reflux by avoiding trigger foods and beverages and implementing eating habits that support digestive health. Certain foods can aggravate symptoms of GERD by producing more stomach acid, relaxing the LES, or irritating the esophageal lining. Examples of well-known triggers include spicy foods, citrus fruits, coffee, alcohol, and chocolate.

Smaller, more frequent meals instead of large ones can also prevent overfilling the stomach and putting pressure on the LES, which reduces the likelihood of acid reflux. In addition to avoiding trigger foods, including non-citrus fruits, vegetables, whole grains, lean proteins (like chicken, fish, and tofu), and low-fat dairy products, can help soothe the esophagus and reduce acid reflux.

Healthy eating practices, like eating slowly, chewing food well, and avoiding lying down right after meals, can help minimize symptoms of gastric reflux disease

(GERD). Keeping a food journal to monitor symptoms and pinpoint personal triggers can help create a customized diet plan for GERD management.

ESSENTIAL GUIDELINES FOR THE GERD DIET

Eating smaller, more frequent meals throughout the day instead of three large ones, which can overload the stomach and increase pressure on the LES, is one of the fundamental principles of the GERD diet, which focuses on reducing acid reflux and relieving symptoms. It also helps prevent stomach contents from refluxing into the esophagus.

Another important rule is to stay away from foods that can aggravate the symptoms of gastro reflux disease (GERD). These foods include spicy foods, citrus fruits and juices, tomatoes and tomato-based products, chocolate, coffee, alcohol, and fatty or fried foods. These foods can cause acid reflux by increasing the production of stomach acid, relaxing the LES, or irritating the lining of the esophagus.

Another important thing to remember is to include foods that are good for you if you have acid reflux disease (GERD). These include non-citrus fruits (bananas, apples, and melons), vegetables (except for tomatoes), whole grains (oatmeal, brown rice, and whole wheat bread), lean proteins (fish, chicken, and tofu), and low-fat dairy products.

In addition, it's critical to be aware of one's eating habits and behaviors. Eating slowly, chewing food well, and avoiding lying down right after meals can all improve digestion and lower the risk of acid reflux. Remaining in a healthy weight range through regular exercise and stress management are also important for maintaining good digestive health and effectively managing symptoms of GERD.

CHAPTER TWO

FOUNDATIONS OF DIET AND GERD

AN OVERVIEW OF SYMPTOMS OF GERD

The symptoms of gastroesophageal reflux disease (GERD) can be very uncomfortable and have a major impact on day-to-day living. GERD patients often experience heartburn, which is a burning sensation in the chest that usually gets worse after eating or sleeping; regurgitation, which is the backflow of stomach contents or acid into the esophagus and leaves a sour or bitter taste in the mouth; dysphagia, or difficulty swallowing; and persistent lumps in the throat. Other symptoms of GERD patients include chronic coughing, hoarseness, and even asthma-like symptoms.

Knowing these symptoms is essential for early detection and successful treatment of GERD. People who recognize these symptoms early on should seek the right medical guidance and make lifestyle adjustments to reduce discomfort and avoid complications.

DIETARY INTERVENTIONS FOR GERD

In addition to reducing stomach acid production and minimizing esophageal irritation, a GERD-friendly diet is crucial for managing the symptoms of gastroesophageal reflux disease (GERD) and promoting overall digestive health.

Acidic and spicy foods, such as citrus fruits, tomatoes, and peppers, can aggravate or trigger acid reflux, so it's important to avoid them. Fried and fatty foods can also relax the lower esophageal sphincter (LES), which allows acid to reflux into the esophagus more readily.

Lean proteins, such as chicken, fish, and tofu, are less likely to cause reflux than red meats; low-fat dairy products provide essential nutrients without contributing to excessive stomach acid production; small, frequent meals spread throughout the day can prevent overeating and reduce pressure on the LES, further mitigating GERD symptoms. On the other hand, incorporating fiber-rich foods, such as whole grains, fruits, and vegetables, supports digestion and helps maintain a healthy weight, which can reduce GERD symptoms.

FOODS NOT TO EAT TO TREAT GERD

To effectively reduce symptoms of gastroparesis (GERD), it is important to avoid foods that are known to aggravate acid reflux. For example, acidic fruits (such as oranges, grapefruits, and lemons) can exacerbate reflux by irritating the esophagus with their high acidity. Tomatoes and tomato-based products (such as sauces and ketchup) are also known to aggravate reflux symptoms due to their high acidity and ability to relax the LES.

Fried and fatty foods like French fries, fried chicken, and greasy burgers contribute to acid reflux by delaying stomach emptying and increasing pressure on the LES. Carbonated beverages, caffeinated drinks like coffee and tea, and alcoholic beverages can also relax the LES and stimulate acid production, exacerbating GERD symptoms. Spicy foods like chili peppers, hot sauces, and curries can irritate the digestive system and promote acid reflux.

By avoiding certain trigger foods and drinks, people with GERD can greatly lessen the frequency and intensity of their episodes, improving their quality of life and ability to manage their illness.

FOODS THAT REDUCE THE SYMPTOMS OF GERD

Eating the right foods can significantly reduce symptoms of gastric reflux disease (GERD) and improve digestive comfort. Non-citrus fruits, such as apples, bananas, and melons, are generally well-tolerated and offer important vitamins and minerals without raising the production of gastric acid. Whole-grain cereals and oatmeal contain fiber, which aids in digestion and helps prevent reflux by encouraging satiety and regulating bowel movements.

Low-fat dairy products like yogurt and skim milk provide calcium and protein without excessive fat that could exacerbate GERD.

Lean proteins like skinless chicken, fish, and tofu provide essential amino acids without triggering reflux symptoms. Vegetables like broccoli, cauliflower, and leafy greens are rich in nutrients and low in acidity, making them excellent choices for those with GERD.

By including these GERD-friendly foods in a balanced diet, people can effectively manage their symptoms and minimize their need for medication. People can also live more comfortably and enhance their overall well-being by emphasizing nutrient-rich foods that support digestive health.

OVERVIEW OF GERD-FRIENDLY COOKING METHODS

Using herbs and mild spices like ginger, parsley, and basil adds flavor without the acidity and heat that can irritate the esophagus. Baking, grilling, and steaming foods instead of frying them reduces the fat content and avoids adding unnecessary calories that can exacerbate GERD symptoms. A diet high in fat can worsen acid reflux symptoms.

Choosing lean meats and cutting fat before cooking helps reduce the chance of reflux; cooking veggies until they are soft but firm preserves their nutrients and lessens the chance of discomforting the digestive tract; and avoiding thick sauces and gravies that are high in fat and acidity can help prevent GERD symptoms from getting worse while still improving the flavor of food.

People can enjoy tasty and nutritious meals that support digestive health and reduce the discomfort associated with GERD by implementing these cooking techniques and making thoughtful food choices. Being proactive in meal preparation can greatly improve quality of life and assist people in managing their condition effectively over an extended period.

CHAPTER THREE

MEAL PLANNING FOR GERD Diet

EVALUATING YOUR EXISTING DIET

It's important to evaluate your current eating habits before beginning a GERD diet plan. This will help you pinpoint triggers and habits that may exacerbate symptoms. To begin, keep a food diary for a week, recording everything you eat and drink as well as any symptoms you experience. Look for trends, such as specific foods or beverages that consistently cause discomfort. You should also pay attention to meal timings and portion sizes, as eating large meals or late at night can exacerbate acid reflux.

Next, assess the nutritional makeup of your diet. Do you get enough fiber, vitamins, and minerals? Do your meals have a lot of fat, spice, or acidity? Knowing these things will help you make the necessary dietary adjustments for a GERD-friendly diet. You can also seek individualized advice from a dietitian or other healthcare provider based on your specific dietary needs and health objectives. With this knowledge in hand, you can proceed to create specific goals for changing your diet to effectively manage your GERD.

DEVELOPING OBJECTIVES FOR YOUR GERD DIET

Achieving success with a GERD diet requires setting specific, attainable goals based on your unique needs and symptoms. For example, if you have nighttime heartburn, your goal might be to stop eating late and make sure you have a gap between dinner and bedtime. If spicy foods make you uncomfortable, your goal might be to cut back on them gradually or find less spicy alternatives.

Setting realistic goals and monitoring your progress will help you stick to your GERD diet plan and achieve improved symptom management over time. It is important to emphasize gradual changes in diet over drastic ones, as sustainable habits are key to the long-term management of GERD. Goals should also address lifestyle factors like maintaining a healthy weight and practicing portion control. You can also incorporate strategies like mindful eating and stress reduction techniques to support your dietary changes.

STRATEGIES FOR MEAL PLANNING

A successful GERD diet begins with effective meal planning. Instead of having three large meals a day, try breaking up your meals into smaller, more frequent portions. This will help you avoid overeating and relieve pressure on your lower esophageal sphincter, which can aggravate reflux.

Include as many GERD-friendly foods as possible, such as lean proteins like chicken and fish, non-citrus fruits and vegetables, whole grains, and low-fat dairy products.

Try cooking with low-fat content, like baking, grilling, or steaming. Steer clear of frying or heavy sauces, which can aggravate symptoms. Use mild or herbaceous spices for flavoring rather than acidic or hot ones.

PLANNING BALANCED MEALS THAT ARE GERD-FRIENDLY: Aim to include a variety of foods from all food groups while avoiding known triggers. To create a balanced meal that supports GERD management, carefully choose ingredients and portion sizes. Begin with a lean protein source, such as grilled chicken or fish, paired with a generous serving of non-citrus vegetables and a small portion of whole grains, such as brown rice or quinoa.

To help ensure a balanced intake and avoid overloading on any one food type that might trigger symptoms, try visualizing your plate as divided into quarters for grains, quarters for vegetables, and quarters for protein. To keep your meals interesting and pleasurable, try experimenting with different recipes and meal combinations that still follow GERD dietary guidelines.

TIPS FOR GROCERY BUYING WITH GERD-FRIENDLY INGREDIENTS

A few smart shopping strategies can make it easier to find GERD-friendly ingredients at the grocery store.

First, plan your meals and create a list based on the recipes you want to make. Next, stay near the perimeter of the store, where fresh produce, lean proteins, and dairy products are usually found. Finally, stay away from the aisles that contain processed foods, snacks, and beverages that could contain triggers like caffeine or carbonation.

Carefully read food labels to identify potential triggers for gastric reflux disease (GERD), such as high-fat content, acidity, or added sugars. Choose whole grains over refined ones. When choosing fruits, choose non-citrus varieties like bananas, apples, and melons. When cooking, add flavorings like ginger, turmeric, and fennel. By shopping carefully and following your list, you can stock your kitchen with GERD-friendly ingredients that support your dietary goals.

RECIPES FOR BREAKFAST

IDEAS FOR GERD-FRIENDLY BREAKFASTS

To effectively manage symptoms, it can be important to find GERD-friendly breakfast ideas. When preparing your morning meals, consider foods that are low in acidity and potential triggers, such as oatmeal with almond milk and bananas, which are low in acidity and provide fiber to aid in digestion. Yogurt with honey and fresh berries is another excellent option, providing probiotics for gut health and antioxidants to combat inflammation. If you like eggs, consider scrambled eggs with spinach and whole-grain toast, which offers a balanced meal with protein and vitamins.

Focusing on nutrient-dense and easily digestible foods will help you start your day feeling nourished and pain-free. Triggers like citrus fruits, spicy foods, and caffeine can exacerbate GERD symptoms. Instead, incorporate soothing options like herbal teas or chamomile tea, which can help to relax the digestive system.

EASY BREAKFAST RECIPES TO FOLLOW

Breakfast can be made with ease when it comes to GERD-friendly recipes. For a protein-packed option, try scrambled eggs with spinach, which is made by whisking eggs, sautéing spinach until it wilts, and serving with whole-grain toast. Another quick idea is a yogurt parfait, which is made by layering plain yogurt with honey and fresh berries in a glass for a colorful and nutritious treat.

Smoothies are a great way to add variation to your diet. Simply blend spinach, banana, almond milk, and a spoonful of almond butter for a creamy, satisfying beverage. These step-by-step recipes are made to be as simple as possible to follow and are specifically formulated to reduce the symptoms of GERD, so you can start your day with ease and comfort.

SIMPLE AND QUICK MORNING MEALS

For people with GERD, quick and simple morning meals can be a lifesaver when you're pressed for time.

Choose low-preparation, gentle-on-the-tongue options like overnight oats, which are simply mixed with almond milk and chilled overnight before being topped with sliced fruit and a sprinkling of nuts in the morning. Another quick and easy option is a smoothie, which is made by blending yogurt, banana, and berries.

To add a savory twist, try avocado toast, which is as easy as mashing an avocado on a slice of whole-grain bread and seasoning with a little salt and pepper. It's a quick and easy breakfast meal that is GERD-friendly, allowing you to maintain a balanced diet without sacrificing taste or nutrition.

HEALTHY SMOOTHIE RECIPE IDEAS

For a hydrating and alkalizing beverage that is rich in vitamins and minerals and easy on the stomach, try blending spinach, cucumber, pineapple, and coconut water into a basic green smoothie. Nutritious smoothie recipes can be a great option for people with GERD, providing a refreshing and easily digestible breakfast option.

A berry smoothie is another delectable option; blend mixed berries, yogurt, and a small amount of almond milk for a creamy, antioxidant-rich breakfast treat. You can also add extra protein and fiber to your smoothies by adding almond butter, chia seeds, or flaxseed meal. These recipes are made to be gentle on the digestive system while still providing vital nutrients to support overall health.

BREAKFAST'S CRITICAL ROLE IN GERD MANAGEMENT

A balanced breakfast helps stabilize blood sugar levels and jump-starts your metabolism, which can prevent overeating later in the day.

For those with GERD, eating smaller, more frequent meals can help reduce symptoms like reflux and heartburn. Recognizing the significance of breakfast in managing GERD is essential for maintaining digestive health and overall well-being.

Making a nutritious breakfast a priority can help you support your body's natural healing processes and improve your quality of life while managing GERD. Low-fat, low-acidity breakfast options can help minimize discomfort and promote healing of the esophagus. Breakfast also offers an opportunity to incorporate foods rich in fiber, vitamins, and minerals, which are essential for digestive health.

RECIPES FOR LUNCH AND DINNER

GERD-SAFE SNACKS FOR LUNCH AND DINNER

Lunch and dinner ideas that are safe for people with gastric reflux disease (GERD) should be low in fat and acidity to minimize the risk of acid reflux. For example, grilled chicken breast with steamed vegetables and brown rice is a low-fat meal that is easy on the stomach and still contains important nutrients. Baked fish with quinoa and roasted vegetables is another great option; fish is easier to digest than red meat, so it's a great choice for people with GERD. Vegetarians can find a satisfying and low-acidity tofu stir-fry with mixed greens and whole-grain noodles. These meals not only help manage GERD symptoms but also provide balanced nutrition for overall health.

APPETIZING AND FILLING MAIN COURSES

Delicious and GERD-friendly entrees require thoughtful ingredient selection and preparation to reduce acid reflux triggers.

For example, a lean beef or turkey burger on a whole grain bun with avocado and a side salad dressed with olive oil and lemon juice is flavorful but light on the stomach because of the lean protein and low acidity. Another option is a vegetable and chickpea curry served over brown rice; curries can be made mild and creamy with coconut milk, which is less likely to trigger heartburn than tomato-based sauces. If you're feeling especially healthy, try a spinach and feta-stuffed chicken breast served over quinoa and steamed asparagus. These entrees demonstrate that GERD-friendly meals can be enjoyable and satisfying.

VEGETABLE-BASED RECIPES TO ALLEVIATE GERD

Since vegetables are generally low in fat and acidity and high in fiber and essential nutrients, they are great options for GERD relief. For example, try a roasted vegetable medley made with bell peppers, zucchini, and carrots seasoned with herbs like thyme and rosemary. Roasting vegetables brings out their flavor without resorting to heavy sauces that can aggravate reflux.

Another great vegetable-based dish is a spinach and mushroom whole grain pasta tossed in a light garlic and olive oil sauce. This dish is comforting but gentle on the stomach, so it's a great choice for those with GERD. Finally, for a quick and nourishing meal, try a mixed greens salad with grilled tofu or shrimp dressed with a lemon vinaigrette dressing.

COOKING TECHNIQUES TO LESSEN GERD SYMPTOMS

It is possible to significantly reduce the symptoms of gastric reflux disease (GERD) by reducing the amount of fat and acidity in meals. Instead of frying, try grilling, baking, or steaming; frying can increase the fat content and make dishes harder to digest.

You can create lean and flavorful protein sources by grilling chicken or fish, or you can bake vegetables with a drizzle of olive oil and herbs to preserve their natural flavors and nutrients. Steaming is another gentle cooking method that retains the nutritional value of foods without adding extra fat. By concentrating on these cooking techniques, you can prepare GERD-friendly meals that are easy on the stomach and promote digestive comfort.

GERD-FRIENDLY SEASONINGS AND FLAVORFUL SAUCES

Making GERD-friendly meals that are still flavorful and enjoyable requires a careful selection of sauces and seasonings. Use herbs like basil, parsley, and cilantro to add freshness and depth to dishes without raising acidity. Lemon juice and vinegar should be used sparingly because they can cause reflux in certain people. Ginger and garlic, on the other hand, can add a kick of flavor without exacerbating GERD symptoms. Cream-based sauces made with low-fat dairy or coconut milk can be a creamy and calming substitute for traditional tomato-based sauces. Experiment with different herb and spice combinations to find flavors that suit your palate while supporting GERD management.

DESSERTS & SNACKS

SNACK OPTIONS THAT ARE GOOD FOR GERD PATIENTS

Selecting healthy snacks for people with gastroesophageal reflux disease (GERD) means avoiding foods that worsen symptoms like acid reflux and heartburn. Choose low-fat and low-acid foods. Fresh fruits, like apples and bananas, are great because of their natural sweetness and low acidity. Whole grain crackers or rice cakes with a small dollop of almond or peanut butter on top provide a satisfying crunch without aggravating GERD symptoms.

Avoid spicy or highly seasoned snacks as they can irritate the esophagus and worsen symptoms of GERD. For those who are craving savory snacks, try low-fat yogurt or cottage cheese with a sprinkle of nuts or seeds for added protein and texture. These dairy options are generally well-tolerated and can help manage hunger between meals without causing discomfort.

SWEETS THAT WON'T MAKE YOUR GERD SYMPTOMS WORSE

When it comes to desserts, choosing foods that are easy on the stomach is key. Fruit salads or smoothies made with non-citrus fruits, such as berries or melons, are light, naturally sweet, and naturally sweet without being acidic. If you're looking for a sweet that feels decadent but won't make you burst into heartburn, try a small piece of dark chocolate or a serving of oatmeal cookies that are low in fat and sugar.

Desserts should be consumed in moderation and portion sizes should be observed to prevent overeating, which can exacerbate GERD symptoms. When baking, substitute ingredients that are known to trigger GERD, such as using applesauce instead of oil or reducing sugar amounts. This approach allows GERD patients to enjoy occasional sweets without sacrificing taste or causing discomfort.

ENERGIZING SNACK IDEAS

Snacks high in nutrients are crucial for managing GERD and maintaining overall health. For example, raw veggies with hummus offer vitamins and fiber without being overly fattening or acidic, and hummus made with chickpeas, olive oil, and garlic is a tasty dip that goes well with cucumber slices, bell pepper strips, or cherry tomatoes.

A handful of mixed nuts or seeds are another nutrient-dense option. Greek yogurt with a drizzle of honey and a sprinkle of nuts or granola is another great choice. Greek yogurt offers probiotics for gut health and protein for satiety. Choose unsalted varieties to avoid excess sodium, which can contribute to bloating and discomfort.

DESSERTS THAT DON'T AGGRAVATE GERD

Desserts that are low in fat and acidity, like angel food cake topped with fresh berries and a dollop of whipped cream, are less likely to trigger reflux than richer, heavier desserts. Making desserts that won't aggravate GERD requires careful ingredient selection and preparation techniques.

Try baked pears or apples with a little honey and cinnamon for a warm treat. These fruits are naturally sweet and high in fiber, which helps with digestion and helps avoid GERD symptoms. When baking, look for recipes that call for whole grains and little added sugar to lessen the chance of experiencing pain after eating.

TIPS FOR PORTION CONTROL IN SNACKING

Controlling portion sizes is essential for avoiding the symptoms of gastric reflux disease (GERD), particularly when snacking. Rather than eating straight from a big bag or container, divide snacks into smaller portions in advance. This will help you avoid overindulging, which can put more pressure on your stomach and possibly cause reflux.

When serving snacks, use small bowls or plates, as this visually signals to the brain that smaller portions are satisfying; also, chew everything thoroughly and enjoy each bite to help with digestion and lower the chance of reflux; and avoid snacking right before bed as this puts more pressure on the lower esophageal sphincter and exacerbates GERD symptoms.

Balancing nutrition and portion control plays a key role in maintaining overall health and minimizing symptoms associated with GERD. Those managing GERD can enjoy tasty treats without discomfort by following these helpful tips and selecting snacks and desserts that are gentle on the digestive system.

DRINKS AND BEVERAGES

RECOGNIZING GERD-FRIENDLY DRINKS

Good GERD (Gastroesophageal Reflux Disease) management depends on the beverages you choose. Low-acidity drinks will not aggravate acid reflux. Non-citrus juices (such as apple, pear, or watermelon juice) are less likely to upset your stomach than acidic juices (like orange or tomato juice). Herbal teas (like chamomile, ginger, and licorice root tea) can also be calming, aiding in digestion and easing the symptoms of reflux. Finally, low-fat milk and coconut water can quench your thirst without making your GERD symptoms worse.

In general, the key is to choose beverages that are gentle on the stomach and won't exacerbate GERD symptoms, promoting comfort and digestive health. Carbonated drinks can aggravate reflux and cause bloating. Alcoholic beverages should also be limited because they relax the lower esophageal sphincter, allowing stomach acid to flow back up into the esophagus. Alkaline water can help neutralize stomach acid and lessen discomfort.

TIPS FOR HYDRATION FOR PEOPLE WITH GERD

It's important to stay hydrated for general health and to help control the symptoms of gastric reflux disease (GERD). Drink small amounts of water throughout the day instead of a large one, which can put pressure on the stomach and exacerbate reflux. It's better to drink water in between meals instead of during meals, as this prevents the stomach acid needed for digestion from becoming diluted. Herbal teas and diluted non-citrus juices can also help stay hydrated without aggravating GERD symptoms.

Caffeine-containing drinks, such as coffee and some teas, should be avoided because they relax the lower esophageal sphincter and cause acid reflux. Instead, choose caffeine-free drinks, like herbal teas or decaffeinated coffee. Having a water bottle on hand all day reminds you to stay hydrated, which promotes overall digestive health and reduces GERD discomfort.

TEAS MADE WITH HERBS TO REDUCE GERD SYMPTOMS

Some herbal teas can help relieve the symptoms of GERD by calming the digestive system and lowering acid reflux. Other teas that help relieve GERD symptoms include ginger tea, which can help with digestion and reduce nausea, chamomile tea, which is well-known for its anti-inflammatory qualities that soothe the lining of the esophagus and reduce discomfort, and licorice root tea, which has natural mucilage properties that can coat the esophagus and relieve heartburn and irritation.

Herbal teas are a safe and gentle way to manage GERD symptoms, offering comfort and support to the digestive system. Brewing herbal teas correctly is important to maximize their medicinal properties; steep them in hot water for the recommended time to fully extract them. Although peppermint tea may be soothing for some digestive issues, it should be avoided by those with GERD as it can relax the lower esophageal sphincter and worsen reflux symptoms.

STEER CLEAR OF TRIGGERING DRINKS

Carbonated beverages, such as soda and sparkling water, introduce gas into the digestive system, potentially causing bloating and increasing pressure on the stomach. Citrus juices, such as orange, grapefruit, and lemon juice, are highly acidic and can irritate the esophagus, leading to heartburn and discomfort. Tomato-based drinks, such as tomato juice and bloody marys, are also acidic and can trigger reflux.

Drinks high in alcohol, especially wine and beer, can relax the lower esophageal sphincter, allowing stomach acid to flow back up into the esophagus and causing heartburn. Caffeinated teas and coffee should be avoided or consumed in moderation because they contain caffeine, which can stimulate acid production and relax the LES. People with GERD can improve their overall quality of life and reduce symptoms by identifying and avoiding these drinks.

MAKING COOL DRINKS WITHOUT CAFFEINE OR CITRUS

The key to making GERD-friendly drinks that are refreshing is to use ingredients that won't aggravate acid reflux. For example, you can make delicious fruit-infused waters or smoothies by blending non-citrus fruits like berries, melons, and apples with almond milk or coconut water. Herbal infusions, like mint-infused water or ginger lemonade (which uses a small amount of ginger for its soothing properties) can offer a refreshing change from traditional citrus-based drinks.

If you like a little fizz, try making sparkling water with slices of cucumber or fresh herbs like mint or basil. Instead of putting citrus fruits straight in your drink, use their zest sparingly to add flavor. Try mixing different fruits and herbs to make refreshing drinks that calm down rather than agitate the digestive system. By making drinks without citrus or caffeine, people with GERD can have tasty options that promote digestive health and reduce discomfort.

CHAPTER FOUR

HANDLING GERD IN PARTICULAR CIRCUMSTANCES

GERD AND EATING OUT: STRATEGIES AND ADVICE

Restaurant navigation for those with GERD requires awareness and planning. Start by looking up GERD-friendly menu items online. Choose dishes that are grilled, baked, or steamed rather than fried or heavily sauced. Ask for sauces and dressings on the side to control portions and steer clear of trigger foods like spicy or acidic foods. Go for smaller portions or share to avoid overeating, which can aggravate symptoms. Eat slowly and chew food thoroughly to aid in digestion and lessen discomfort. Finally, sip water in between bites to help manage your GERD.

Planning and making thoughtful choices can make dining out with GERD enjoyable and symptom-free. When dining out, communication is essential. Tell your server about your dietary restrictions due to GERD and ask for modifications, such as asking for whole-grain alternatives or replacing fatty sides with vegetables. Stay away from carbonated beverages and alcohol and stick to herbal teas or water instead. After the meal, resist the urge to lie down right away and take a leisurely walk to aid in digestion.

TRAVELING WHILE KEEPING YOUR GERD DIET IN CHECK

Preparing ahead of time will help you travel with GERD and avoid discomfort. Pack GERD-friendly snacks, such as nuts, seeds, and whole-grain crackers, for easy access during flights or road trips. Look for GERD-friendly options at local grocery stores and restaurants, such as lean proteins, vegetables, and whole grains. If your GERD flares up, think about bringing along over-the-counter antacids or prescription medications.

Planning and sticking to a consistent diet and routine will make traveling with GERD easier and more enjoyable. Regular meals and snacks will help prevent overeating, which can exacerbate symptoms of GERD.

If dining out isn't an option, opt for accommodations with kitchenettes or mini-fridges to make easy, homemade meals. Remain hydrated with water and avoid caffeine and alcohol, which can exacerbate acid reflux. Walking and yoga are gentle activities that can help with digestion and reduce stress, which is a common cause of GERD symptoms.

GET-TOGETHERS AND GERD-FRIENDLY DECISIONS

When attending social events with GERD, it's important to carefully consider what to eat and drink to avoid discomfort. Before the event, let the host know about your dietary needs and offer to bring something lighter. Some ideas are grilled vegetables, lean proteins, and salads without heavy dressings or acidic dressings. Citrus fruits, tomatoes, and spicy dishes are trigger foods; instead, go for plain options or ask for modifications.

Instead of concentrating only on food during social gatherings, concentrate on mingling with others. Pace yourself while eating, taking small bites, and chewing thoroughly to aid in digestion and reduce reflux. Drink water or herbal teas instead of alcohol or carbonated beverages, as these can exacerbate symptoms. After eating, partake in light physical activity, such as dancing or taking a stroll, to aid in digestion and ease discomfort.

HOW TO CELEBRATE AND HANDLE HOLIDAYS

To maximize enjoyment and minimize discomfort, it is necessary to plan for holiday celebrations with GERD. Start by looking over menus in advance and noting GERD-friendly options like roasted meats, steamed vegetables, and whole-grain sides. You can also prepare meals at home with non-trigger ingredients so you have healthy options to traditional holiday fare. If you are attending a gathering, let the host know about your dietary restrictions and offer to bring a dish that meets your needs.

Planning and making informed choices can help make holiday celebrations with GERD symptom-free and enjoyable.

Practice portion control and refrain from overindulging in rich, fatty foods or sweets, which can exacerbate acid reflux. Choose smaller servings and take your time to savor each bite, chewing thoroughly to aid in digestion. Avoid lying down right after meals; instead, engage in light activities like playing outdoor games or taking a leisurely walk.

HANDLING GERD IN HIGH-STRESS SITUATIONS

To maintain overall health and digestive health during stressful times, managing GERD requires a holistic approach. You should prioritize eating regular meals and snacks throughout the day to prevent overeating, which can cause discomfort and reflux.

You should also include foods high in fiber, such as fruits, vegetables, and whole grains, in your diet to support digestion and lower the risk of acid reflux. Finally, you should practice stress-reduction techniques, such as deep breathing, meditation, or yoga, to minimize triggers that can exacerbate GERD symptoms.

Limit your intake of caffeine and alcohol during stressful times as these can aggravate symptoms of GERD. Maintain optimal digestion by staying hydrated with water and herbal teas. Make sure you have access to prescription medications or over-the-counter antacids to relieve symptoms as needed. Get regular exercise, such as walking or swimming, to improve digestion and lower stress levels. Create a regular sleep schedule to support overall digestive health and minimize reflux at night. By emphasizing self-care and developing healthy habits, managing GERD during stressful times can be manageable and supportive of long-term wellness.

CHAPTER FIVE

LIFESTYLE SUGGESTIONS TO REDUCE GERD

THE VALUE OF EXERCISE IN THE MANAGEMENT OF GERD

Exercise is a key component of managing Gastroesophageal reflux disease (GERD) because it improves overall digestive health and helps manage weight. It also improves digestion by improving the movement of food through the digestive tract, which lowers the risk of acid reflux. Exercises such as yoga, jogging, or walking strengthens the muscles that support the digestive system, which helps reduce GERD symptoms like heartburn and regurgitation.

Excess weight can put pressure on the abdomen and stomach, increasing the risk of acid reflux. Exercise also helps you maintain a healthy weight, which is important for controlling GERD. By adding physical activity to your daily routine, you can improve your overall health and manage your weight. It's important to choose activities that you enjoy and can stick with over time, as consistency is key to reaping the benefits of exercise for managing GERD.

And last, exercise reduces stress, which is another factor that exacerbates GERD symptoms. Reducing stress levels through exercise also helps to indirectly alleviate symptoms like discomfort and chest pain. All things considered, including regular physical activity in your routine is a proactive step towards effectively managing GERD and enhancing your quality of life.

STRATEGIES FOR STRESS REDUCTION IN GERD PATIENTS

Stress management is important for people with GERD because stress can aggravate or cause symptoms like acid reflux and heartburn. Progressive muscle relaxation, deep breathing exercises, and mindfulness meditation are good ways to reduce stress because they help relax the body and mind and lower the amount of stress hormones that can aggravate digestive problems.

Regular exercise, like yoga or tai chi, can also help lower stress levels and encourage relaxation.

Hobbies or other enjoyable activities can also act as a diversion from everyday stressors, which can enhance your mental health and lessen the symptoms of GERD.

Prioritizing self-care and making time for relaxation each day are crucial. Keeping a regular sleep schedule and getting enough sleep can also help manage stress and alleviate GERD symptoms. By incorporating these stress-reduction strategies into your everyday routine, you can reduce the negative effects of stress on your digestive system and improve your overall quality of life.

GERD AND SLEEP HYGIENE

A regular sleep schedule, a calming nighttime routine, and optimizing your sleep environment are all important components of maintaining good sleep hygiene, which is crucial for managing the symptoms of gastroparesis reflux disease (GERD). Reducing nighttime reflux symptoms can also be achieved by avoiding large meals and acidic foods close to bedtime.

Sleeping on your left side may also help relieve GERD symptoms by keeping the stomach below the esophagus, reducing the likelihood of acid reflux. You can also try raising the head of your bed slightly with bed risers or using a wedge pillow to help prevent stomach acid from refluxing into the esophagus while you sleep.

Reducing alcohol and caffeine consumption, especially in the evening, helps improve the quality of sleep and lessen GERD symptoms during the night. Before bed, try deep breathing exercises or guided imagery to help you relax and fall asleep.

Your daily routine can be optimized to improve digestive health and lessen the frequency and intensity of GERD symptoms by implementing these sleep hygiene measures.

KEEPING A HEALTHY WEIGHT TO MANAGE GERD

A balanced diet rich in fruits, vegetables, and whole grains will help you reach and maintain a healthy weight, which is important for treating the symptoms of GERD because being overweight puts strain on the abdomen and aggravates acid reflux.

Portion control and mindful eating are also key strategies for managing both weight and acid reflux disease (GERD). Eating slowly and avoiding large meals can help minimize the risk of acid reflux and reduce the likelihood of overeating. It's also helpful to recognize and steer clear of foods that can aggravate acid reflux symptoms, such as citrus fruits, spicy foods, and caffeine.

Regular physical exercise can help you maintain a healthy weight and lessen the frequency of GERD symptoms. It can also assist in weight management and promote digestive health. Some enjoyable activities to include in your routine are walking, swimming, or cycling.

You may effectively control your GERD and enhance your overall quality of life by concentrating on reaching and maintaining a healthy weight with a balanced diet and frequent exercise.

DAILY ROUTINES TO ENCOURAGE GERD-FREE LIVING

Maintaining a GERD-free lifestyle requires incorporating daily habits that support digestive health. While eating smaller, more frequent meals throughout the day can help prevent overeating and lower the risk of acid reflux, it's crucial to wait at least two to three hours after eating before lying down or going to bed.

Avoiding smoking and consuming as little alcohol as possible can also help manage the symptoms of GERD because they weaken the lower esophageal sphincter and increase acid reflux. Drinking lots of water throughout the day can also support digestive function and lower the risk of acid reflux.

Adding fiber-rich foods to your diet, such as whole grains, fruits, and vegetables, can also improve digestive health and lessen symptoms of GERD. Maintaining excellent posture, such as sitting upright during and after meals, can encourage healthy digestion and minimize strain on the abdomen.

You can enhance your overall digestive health and effectively manage your GERD symptoms by including these daily activities into your routine. Since consistency is essential to living a GERD-free lifestyle, it's critical to prioritize these behaviors as part of your daily routine for long-term symptom relief.

CHAPTER SIX

RECIPES FOR PARTICULAR EVENTS

RECIPES FOR PARTIES AND GATHERINGS THAT ARE GERD-FRIENDLY

Party planning for people with gastric reflux disease (GERD) requires careful menu planning that is delicious but easy on the stomach. Begin your event with light appetizers like grilled vegetable skewers or cucumber and hummus bites; these won't make you feel queasy.

main courses, think about satisfying dishes like seafood paella made with fresh ingredients and mild spices, or grilled chicken with quinoa and steamed vegetables.

Plan and choose carefully selected ingredients to create a party menu that everyone will enjoy while avoiding GERD symptoms. For beverages, serve mocktails with fresh fruit juices or infused water instead of alcohol and carbonated drinks.

For dessert, choose GERD-friendly treats like fruit salad with a dollop of Greek yogurt or a light angel food cake with fresh berries.

HOLIDAY MENUS THAT DON'T MAKE YOUR GERD WORSE

Holiday feasts can be made GERD-friendly by making simple substitutions. Traditional holiday menus can be made GERD-friendly by starting with a creamy carrot ginger soup made with almond milk instead of heavy cream for the soup course. Roast turkey or baked salmon seasoned with herbs and served with roasted sweet potatoes and steamed green beans make excellent main course choices.

Holiday meals can be enjoyed without worrying about GERD flare-ups by focusing on fresh, whole foods and avoiding heavy fats and spices. Some ideas for side dishes are quinoa pilaf with roasted vegetables or fresh spinach salad with strawberries and light vinaigrette. Desserts can be tricky, but options like poached pears with honey and cinnamon or a fruit tart with a gluten-free crust and dairy-free whipped topping can satisfy sweet cravings without causing discomfort.

PREPARING FOOD FOR VISITORS WITH GERD CONCERNS

When cooking for guests with GERD, it's important to plan so that everyone feels comfortable throughout the meal. For starters, try crudites with a yogurt-based dip or a cool gazpacho made with ripe tomatoes and cucumber. For the main course, try flavorful but mildly marinated grilled chicken or tofu skewers served with quinoa and steamed broccoli on the side.

As you plan the menu, get to know your guests' triggers and preferences. Steer clear of dishes that feature heavy creams, fried foods, or spicy ingredients. Instead, go for lighter preparations that highlight lean proteins, fresh vegetables, and whole grains. For dessert, think about serving a fresh fruit platter or a light sorbet made with natural fruit juices. With careful thought and preparation, you can create a wonderful meal that suits everyone's dietary needs, including those with GERD.

ENJOYING YOURSELF WITHOUT LOSING YOUR DIET

Enjoying special occasions without sacrificing flavor or enjoyment is possible with GERD management. Start with appetizers such as watermelon and feta salad or bruschetta with diced tomatoes and basil on whole grain bread. For the main course, try satisfying recipes like grilled shrimp skewers marinated in citrus or a turkey burger with avocado and lettuce on a whole wheat bun.

Instead of alcohol and sugary drinks, serve mocktails with herbal infusions or fresh fruit purees; for dessert, present a fruit platter with yogurt dip or a gluten-free apple crisp made with oats and almond flour. By choosing your ingredients carefully and limiting your portion sizes, you can celebrate guilt-free without aggravating your GERD symptoms.

DESSERT IDEAS FOR SPECIAL OCCASIONS THAT WON'T SET OFF GERD

It's surprising how easy it is to find GERD-friendly dessert options for special occasions. Some ideas are to serve Greek yogurt, fresh berries, and granola layers in a berry parfait, or make a chia seed pudding with almond milk, sliced bananas, and honey for a crunchy and satisfying treat that won't make your reflux flare up.

A delicious alternative is a crustless pumpkin pie made with coconut milk and sweetened with agave nectar or stevia. If you're more of a baked person, try making a flourless chocolate cake using almond flour and cocoa powder, sweetened with a little honey or maple syrup. Desserts low in fat and acidity allow you to enjoy sweets without having to worry about your GERD symptoms spoiling the festivities.

CHAPTER SEVEN

COMMON QUESTIONS AND CONCERNS

CONTROLLING GERD SYMPTOMS WITHOUT MEDICATIONS

If you want to manage your GERD symptoms without taking medication, you need to make deliberate dietary and lifestyle changes to reduce discomfort and the frequency of acid reflux episodes.

One of the most important strategies is to change the way you eat. You should eat smaller, more frequent meals to prevent overloading your stomach, which can cause reflux. You should also recognize and stay away from foods that make your symptoms worse, like spicy foods, citrus fruits, and caffeine.

Maintaining a healthy weight is also essential for managing GERD. Being overweight puts strain on your abdomen and exacerbates reflux; therefore, eating a balanced diet and getting regular exercise can help.

Raising the head of your bed by 6 to 8 inches can also lessen the symptoms of reflux at night by preventing stomach acid from flowing back into your esophagus while you sleep.

Finally, stress management is critical because stress aggravates GERD symptoms. Deep breathing exercises, meditation, and yoga are some techniques that help lower stress levels and enhance general health. By regularly putting these lifestyle changes into practice, people can frequently significantly reduce GERD symptoms without using medication alone.

HANDLING EPISODES OF GERD

Managing flare-ups of gastric reflux disease (GERD) involves both short-term measures and long-term management plans. In the event of a flare-up, avoid foods and drinks that can aggravate symptoms, such as alcohol, caffeine, spicy foods, and fatty foods; instead, choose smaller, blander meals that are easier on the digestive tract.

In addition to drinking lots of water, taking over-the-counter antacids can help dilute stomach acid and wash it back down into the stomach. However, it's important to follow the dosage instructions carefully and avoid using antacids as a long-term solution.

Long-term relief from acid reflux during sleep can be achieved by keeping a food diary, which can help identify specific triggers that cause flare-ups and help you avoid them in the future. Other measures that may be necessary to treat acid reflux during sleep include elevating the head of your bed and avoiding lying down right after meals.

LONG-TERM GERD MANAGEMENT TECHNIQUES

Maintaining a GERD-friendly diet, which includes avoiding trigger foods like spicy and acidic foods as well as carbonated beverages, is essential to the long-term management of GERD. Consuming smaller, more frequent meals and including foods that are high in fiber and low in fat will help reduce the frequency and severity of symptoms.

Maintaining a healthy weight through diet and exercise is important for long-term GERD management, as excess weight can put pressure on the abdomen and exacerbate reflux symptoms. Regular physical activity not only helps with weight management but also lowers stress levels, which can exacerbate GERD symptoms.

Apart from that, giving up alcohol and smoking can also help people with GERD symptoms because they both relax the lower esophageal sphincter, which makes it easier for stomach acid to reflux into the esophagus. People can also improve their overall digestive health by giving up alcohol and smoking and moderating their intake of both of these substances.

TIPS FOR PATIENTS WITH RECENTLY DIAGNOSED GERD

For those who have recently been diagnosed with gastroesophageal reflux disease (GERD), the first step in managing symptoms and enhancing the quality of life is education about GERD and its triggers. This includes knowing which foods and drinks make symptoms worse and which lifestyle choices—such as smoking and binge drinking—may aggravate reflux.

Maintaining a food diary can help identify specific triggers and patterns, empowering patients to make educated dietary choices that reduce symptoms. Eating smaller, more frequent meals and avoiding trigger foods like citrus fruits, tomatoes, and caffeine are essential components of a GERD-friendly diet.

Apart from dietary modifications, it's critical to maintain a healthy weight through diet and exercise. Being overweight can aggravate GERD symptoms by placing pressure on the abdomen, which increases reflux. Frequent physical activity helps manage weight and lowers stress, both of which can help relieve symptoms.

Finally, seeking advice and treatment options from medical professionals who specialize in digestive health, such as gastroenterologists or dietitians, can offer tailored guidance.

Newly diagnosed patients can better control their symptoms and improve their long-term prognosis by managing their GERD early on.

FREQUENTLY ASKED QUESTIONS REGARDING THE DIET FOR GERD

Managing acid reflux through dietary modifications often raises questions and concerns, one of which is whether spicy foods are allowed.

Spicy foods, like acidic foods like tomatoes and citrus fruits, are known to trigger symptoms of acid reflux disease and should be avoided or consumed in moderation.

One more frequently asked question concerns caffeine's effect on gastroesophageal reflux disease (GERD). As caffeine relaxes the lower esophageal sphincter, it makes it easier for stomach acid to reflux into the esophagus. To effectively manage the symptoms of GERD, limit or avoid caffeine-containing beverages, such as coffee, tea, and soda.

Another thing to be concerned about for people with GERD is alcohol consumption. In addition to its potential to relax the lower esophageal sphincter and increase stomach acid production, alcohol should be consumed in moderation; some people may find that they can tolerate alcohol better in smaller amounts than others.

Many people are curious about how dietary lipids affect the management of gastric reflux disease (GERD). Eating high-fat meals can cause delayed stomach emptying and raise the risk of acid reflux. Choosing low-fat foods and avoiding fried and fatty foods can help alleviate symptoms and enhance overall comfort in the digestive system.

Eating smaller meals throughout the day and avoiding large meals right before bedtime can reduce nighttime reflux and prevent excessive pressure on the stomach.

www.ingramcontent.com/pod-product-compliance
Lightning Source LLC
Chambersburg PA
CBHW071842210526
45479CB00001B/248